SICK OF IT

Be Sexy, Healthy, Fit & FREE without the stress of Diet and Exercise

Romi "The Mighty Singh" Gill

SICK OF IT

This book is dedicated to my parents for teaching me the value of hard work and living an honest life while helping those in need. Also a shout out to my brother for supporting me in good and bad times. And to my first lady who was a missing piece in my life.

Table of Contents

Foreword by Melissa Krivachek

Many people mistakenly believe that dieting and cardio is a requirement to losing weight. It isn't. In fact our bodies define us; they represent our unique characters. Yet they test and challenge us to take care of our greatest lifelong asset. Our success in fitness does not lie in taking away our favorite foods forever or engaging in less than desirable exercises. It does lie in how we deal with what we have, and how we transform our unique body into the body of our dreams.

We have the capacity to change the physiology of our body, to create more confidence in every area of our life. This requires treating our body like a temple and making it a top priority. To do this however, it's essential that we become aware of what our body not only wants but needs to keep it in peak condition. Because, it is the only thing we are born and die with and it's the one thing that enhances both our lives and longevity.

The principles in this book act as navigational tools to help guide you along in your weight loss journey. They are like a set of operating instructions to get you from where you are to the body of your dreams. While helping you remain stress free and calm along the way. As you become thinner you will gain clarity and confidence to accomplish everything you want and more.

In this extraordinary book fitness fanatic Romi Gill who's been in love and competed in the industry for more than a decade explains why fitness is not your enemy, but rather your friend if you allow it to be. He reminds us that our bodies are powerful tools that can work for us or against us at any given moment. We have a choice. We can learn to fuel our body like a Ferrari or let it deteriorate like a beat up truck.

As you read this book reflect on your goals and you will see that despite where you are right now, you too can have the body of your dreams! God Bless.

SICK OF IT

Preface

"Get your fat ass out of bed and do something with your life", she said.

She didn't use those exact words, but that's what she meant. Mothers can be blatantly honest to our face because they have known us since birth. I had lost all motivation when I was at a low point and had to depend on my parents for money. More on this story later.

In this book I share my experience of going from a bodybuilder with a life of average success to a lifeless loser and then back to a life of no limits and endless motivation. At this low point I had gone from having a body to kill for to an unsightly fat body coupled with a very negative mindset with no hope and passion.

I was sick of all the bullshit in my life, I was sick of living a "prescription life" where we have to do what we were told, we have to eat tasteless food and do endless exercise to stay fit, I was sick of lying, I was sick of not being able to express myself, I was sick of sugar coating things to be politically correct. It felt like I was living in a futuristic movie where the world is run by robots and humans don't have much freedom and are treated like slaves.

After a proverbial kick in the ass by my mom, I got up and said "F*CK IT!" I made the decision to make a positive change in my life.

That's when I started on an awesome journey that brought me here today. The new Romi lives a life full of passion with no limits or conditions. A life in which

Romi does what he wants and eats what he wants without worrying about pleasing or offending others.

I found the secret to live life to the fullest where I am in control. The reason I am sharing this is because I come across a lot of people in person and over Facebook who are also stuck in life with no hope, and my experience can help them move forward. You can also use my secret to become happy and healthy.

Like rapper Drake said, "Started from the bottom, now we here."

I want to thank my coach Melissa Krivachek who helped me stop procrastinating and go from a Personal Trainer to becoming a motivational speaker and lighting a fire under my ass (holding me accountable) to write this book.

Romi Gill

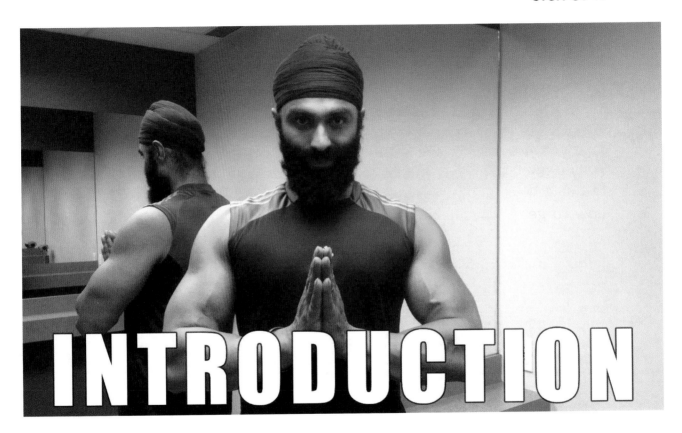

You are reading this book because you don't have the body you want and you are worried about your long-term health and well-being.

This book will teach you how to be healthy while maintaining a healthy weight, and having fun going from the way you are now to getting the body you want.

You are going to like me because, just like you, I also want the fast and easy way of doing things. I believe there's more than one way to lose fat. I will show you how to get the body you want, without going through the traditional methods which you hate, and have fun while doing it.

I was brainwashed into doing what's popular and trendy. But then I woke up and took control of my mind and my life. I was a follower, and then I became a leader who leads by example. I don't follow the rules of society that teach us to accept and live a shitty life (A life full of limiting and negative beliefs and no freedom). I do what makes me a better person, makes me happy and makes me a good role model that people can look up to.

I am blunt, I am politically incorrect, I make my own rules (no, I don't break the law), and live life to the fullest. My life's purpose is to bring happiness and positive energy into other people's lives. I have this excessive positive energy given to me and I love sharing it with others. I practice what I preach. My methods are unusual but my bullshit-free approach produces results.

I want to change the world by helping people become good role models who go out and spread the positive message.

"Be good, teach others to be good and inspire them to infect other people with positivity." **RomiVirus**.

^ Tweet that shit.

In this book I will teach you how to love yourself, how to be sexy, healthy, fit and free of negative energy and limiting thoughts. BOOM.

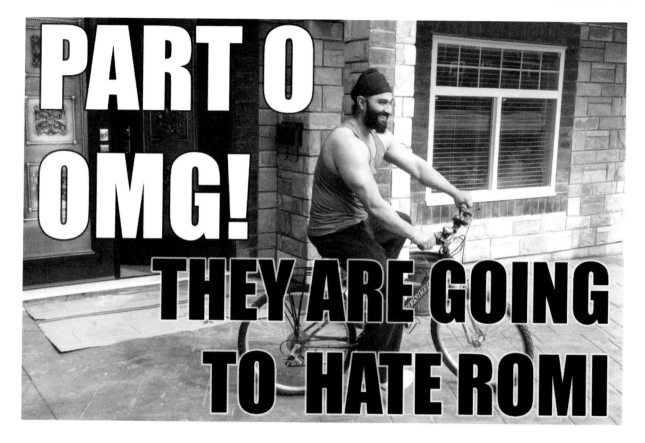

I am going to be hated by the following groups of people -

- Authors
- Doctors
- Personal Trainers &
- Athletes

Authors will hate me because I am writing this book in conversation style – it's like I am telling a story to a friend (and yes, you are my friend – after all you bought my book, haha).

There are no chapters, you should expect bad grammar, spelling mistakes and poems that don't make sense, and words everybody uses while texting and talking on social media websites like "haha", "omg", "lol" (it means Laugh Out Loud) and "BOOM". I might use profanity as well, be warned. I am different, this book is different – deal with it.

Disclaimer: If you are easily offended **GTFO**, go read a comic book or go to the Disney world website, my language might be too strong for you. **You Mad Bro?**

Doctors will hate me because I will not stop you from eating carbs, fat and all the other shit you want to eat that they tell you not to.

Question: How many fat doctors can you think of?

*Hey, **do you ever wonder why** over 60% of hospital staff is overweight? I am not going to tell you, go to an overweight doctor or a nurse and ask them. (be prepared to run, we don't want you to die, haha.)*

Because my methods are different I am going to get a lot of hate from doctors, traditional personal trainers and traditional athletes who are stuck in their ways. I don't care what they think – all I care about is getting you results.

I don't care how you get results – exercise, diet, pills, water manipulation, etc.. You must do what it takes to become healthy and fit. There are doctors who will tell you everything is unsafe and yet these are the professionals who keep you fat.

Listen up:
*"Too much Body fat is not healthy, it wasn't healthy a hundred years ago, it's not healthy now and it's not going to be healthy in a hundred years! – **Coach Romi Gill**"*

^ Tweet that shit!

My Jamaican friend, who loves big girls, always says this about them (say this in a Jamaican accent): *"Man, dem big gals keep you warm in winter and give you shade in summer."* lol

STOP LAUGHING, OMG You are so mean, Shame on you!! It's not funny, and definitely not a good reason to stay overweight, lol.

If someone's advice is keeping you fat, run in the opposite direction as fast as you can. Especially, if they are fat themselves.

Most **Personal Trainers** and **Athletes** are used to strict diets and daily exercise and this is what they preach. Their approach definitely works, **but clearly it's not working for you**. They hate me because I don't force you to stop eating junk food! They hate me more because I am a competitive bodybuilder and I live this lifestyle close to my competition, but for the rest of the year I live life, lol.

I am very goofy and I use humor and sarcasm a lot. Get used to terms like "Fitness Warriors", "RomiVirus", "RomiMagic", "BOOM", ans poems that intentionally don't rhyme, for example:

"Roses are red,

Violets are blue…

This is Romi's poem,

It NEVER Rhymes. Thank you."

This book offers a solution that **GUARANTEES** results. There is no boring stuff like case studies, scientific studies, and references to websites, books etc. (OMG I am falling asleep already). If you are into all that this book is not for you!

Some of you are probably thinking "OMG! *this guy is so dumb, but he is very entertaining and GUARANTEES results, and he is super cool. I might as well read his shit. I paid money to buy his book"*. My response "If words could kill… never mind. I am glad words can't kill me, lol."

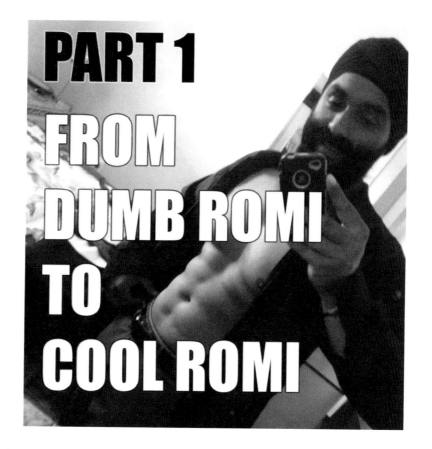

Romi's sad little story

This book is a result of over thirteen years of my personal experience in fitness and endless frustrating hours to get hundreds of people to get in the shape they want (weight loss, weight gain, getting toned, sports performance, or 6pac abs).

As a competitive bodybuilder and a personal trainer I was programmed to make people eat the usual strict tasteless diet and do endless cardio to lose weight. **People like you were so mean**, they never ate 6 healthy meals a day and never did the recommended daily cardio. Was it too much to ask for?

I could not understand why people are willing to stay out of shape, willing to accept the risk of disease and not give up junk food when all doctors and personal trainers were preaching this. Hundreds of diet plans for clients and friends with hundreds of hours of customizing to cater to each person, went to waste. I used to get frustrated and think *"OMG! I am such a sweet guy, how could they break my heart?"*

One day (in 2006) I ended up at a seminar hosted by a "pyramid-scheme" company where I picked by a book by Tony Robbins called "Unlimited Power". I read it and BOOM, I was hooked. I started my self-development journey. I started learning about the human mind, psychology, and studied things like propaganda, mind control, NLP and tricks used by corporations and politicians to brainwash us using the media. I felt like a fool for not knowing these techniques before. I could have used them myself for my career and to help other people succeed.

Watch out, if you start acting like a chicken, it would mean you are under Romi's Hypnotic spell. HAHAHA (Romi's evil laugh). And to break the spell you will have to **buy another book** for a friend and then **my second book**. Thank You, Sir!

The years 2010 and 2011 were full of stress for me - I had given up bodybuilding and had no motivation in life. I had become a Zombie (and no, I did not go around killing people, lol).

I lost my job and was not able to find a job for 2 years I feared I was going to be homeless. I was up to my ears in credit card debt. I did not know how I was going to pay it off. My family loves me, they paid off my debt and I became dependent on them.

It is the worst thing that could happen to a grown man, who is physically and mentally fit, but is not able to earn a living and is dependent on his parents (especially when I was brought up in a family who believed in working hard).

NOTE: Trust me, being "forever alone" is not the worst thing for a man, lol.

I was born in the Sikh faith that originated from the North Indian state of Punjab. Like most other people, I also saw religion as a cult and a scheme to make money. When I was at my lowest point in life I decided to blame God.

To my surprise I was able find God so fast and escape the bullshit of religious leaders, politicians and other evil people involved in religion who brainwash innocent people. Sikhi (The Sikh faith) is a simple lifestyle where the main focus is connecting to God through prayer, humility and good deeds thus charging your mind with positive energy. In Sikhi you are also taught to become a warrior and stand up against injustice.   Being a bodybuilder, this was not a difficult task. I had a lot of ego, which I was able to eliminate following the principles of Sikhi.

"A real Warrior is the one who fights his or her inner demons (anger, ego, lust, greed, and attachment)."

^ Tweet that shit

My life completely changed within a matter of months, I got back on my feet, I became positive, and I found the purpose of my life which was to bring happiness and positivity in other people's lives, especially the ones who have lost all hope.

I became a new person. Ego, anger, hate, fear, and negativity were gone for the most part. I felt incredibly empowered with a divine energy because I learnt that God isn't sitting somewhere in the sky, he is within each one of us. With the absence of ego and fear, I started seeing the world in a different way.

I added the title "**The Mighty Singh**" to my name on Facebook. Singh is a Punjabi word for lion. All Sikh men are given this identity (and middle name) by our Guru. He taught us to be brave, and stand up to all types of bullying and defend others. A true Sikh man (and women who are given the name Kaur) will give his life to protect you.

Although I was positive, I decided not to train because I thought building muscle will give me a bigger ego. I was taught a lesson when two of my friends (Babbar Singh and Surjit Singh) approached me at the Gurdwara (Sikh Temple) and asked me to train them.

I said, "Are you blind? Look at me, I am FAT, how can I make you lose weight, when I look like shit!" They believed in me and brought me back to the gym.

"You can take a bodybuilder out of the Gym, but you can't take the Gym out of a bodybuilder. Once a bodybuilder, always a bodybuilder." – Coach Romi Gill

"We are all given unique gifts, talents and skills. We must use them positively to make this world a better place." – Coach Romi Gill

^ Tweet that shit.

My skill was my ability to teach people. Teach them how to be mentally strong and how to take care of their body and health. I decided to start giving.

Psychology and spirituality gave me so much mental strength that I was able to realize how much we are brainwashed to follow blindly what politicians, corporations and the media feeds us.

I got **"SICK OF IT"** and decided to take control of my life. I stopped watching TV and stopped listening to the radio because of all the negative shit promoted on both.

Another life changing event happened around 2007 when I was chatting up a girl. I was trying to be cool by showing off how much I know about Fitness and how I can make any girl look "hot".

Before I continue you must know one thing about me – I was a ladies man!

OK, OK, OK, I lied - I used to get friendzoned all the time. But that's what I told myself and all the girls I talked to. Now, don't be mean, be nice to your coach because you are under Romi's spell, lol.

Oh come on, don't I get an E for Effort?

She said, "Mr. Bodybuilder: what's the point of killing yourself in the gym every day when you can't enjoy the food of your liking".

I was really pissed off. I know what you are all thinking. **No, I did not slap her!**

Seriously, her comment made me think but I didn't take any action. I said to myself, "what does this chick know about fitness."

I had a clever comeback. Even though she was not fat, I said, "RIGHT! If I did that, I'd end up looking like you, a Potato, haha". Needless to say, she told me to get lost.

I competed again in 2012 but I hated every minute of dieting for my competition. I was **"SICK OF IT"** – sick of dieting, sick of pretending to enjoy tasteless food day in and day out. I said to myself, **"F*ck it**! I am going to eat whatever I want, whenever I want and I am not going to pretend to be miserable". That's when I found the secret to stress-free health and happiness for life.

I decided to change my training and the diet of my clients and BOOM people started to get in shape without being grumpy and hating me.

IQ Test: Mary's father has 5 daughters – Nana, Nana, Nini, and Nono. Who's the 5th daughter?
Answer: Mary. Gotcha! This proves you have been brainwashed, lol.

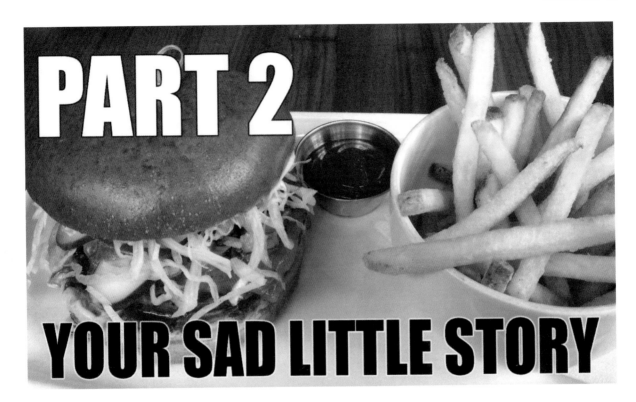

Something tells me that you are like me, lazy, err I mean a cool person who wants an easy way out.

Maybe you are also "**SICK OF IT**" - sick of not having a choice, sick of feeling bad, sick of people judging you, sick of not living the life you want, and sick of all the other bullshit that makes you unhappy. And most of all, Sick of being a slave.

You are going to listen to me because in the past I have been stupid, fat, stressed (what most people call depressed), an ego-maniac, and yet I overcame all of that and made a positive change to become the person I am today, FREE, healthy and fit. Ladies also tell me I am very attractive. I am not lying. OK, FINE – At least one girl, my first lady, thinks I am attractive and that's good enough for me.

My secret formula is guaranteed to work. And 'The Mighty Singh' is going to help you become a better you.

THE COLD HARD TRUTH

You probably won't admit it but you are worried about the way you look and if you, like most, don't have the physical appearance that our society has projected to be "sexy" you are stressed out and always looking for easy shortcuts to get the shape you want. Don't worry, you are in good hands.

You want a simple and fun way to live a healthy and happy life, right?

If you agree, give me a "BOOM".

Come on, say "BOOOOOOOOM."

<u>If you do, you are allowed to have a cookie guilt-free</u> :)

THIS IS A MESSED UP SOCIETY

Society/Media tells us how we are supposed to look, how we are supposed to live our life, how we are supposed to eat, and how we are supposed to raise our kids, how we are supposed to educate them, tells us what to think etc.

WHO MADE THEM THE BOSS?

They call this "the norm", the normal way of doing things. The media always tries to dumb us down to sell us more products and services and to make us more complacent.

Negative programming creates low self-esteem, negative and/or limiting mindset, bad self-image, lack of focus and ambition, and on top of that, we are surrounded by unmotivated and negative people. Ambitious and hard-working people are called "Crazy", a bad/mediocre life is acceptable, and we must not say what hurts other people's feelings. Want the brutal honest truth? We are like sheep and must of us follow what others are doing because otherwise we risk being left alone or not fitting in.

Some of you probably think the same way that I used to think, "I don't give a shit about society, I live my life the way I want to live it."

But at the same time you fear what society thinks of you, you have "what would people say" syndrome!

This society ridicules people who become vegetarian and accepts or forgives people who drink, smoke or do recreational drugs. WTF is that?

QUESTION: Would you stand in the middle of a busy mall and get someone to take your picture while you are doing something silly? I know I will, and I have made people take pictures of me "posing" in public all the time.

If your answer is no, or, "that's stupid/silly" it means you have "what would people say" syndrome. We are going to change that.

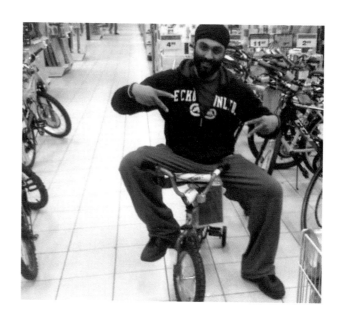

Check this out, do you run into situations when people say something stupid like "blah blah blah... they say opposites attract etc etc etc". I shoot back, "THEY? Who are they? Tell me who, let me have a chat with them". Of course, nobody knows who "they" are, other than "other people".

For the record, I am still looking for "them", if you find them let me know.

You are nothing but a Robot – not the intelligent kind, lol, but the one with reduced functionality. When you decide to break free of the brainwashing and become human again, you are looked down upon because that's they you start making decisions for yourself.

"Some people are so negative, when you put them in a dark room they start to develop" – Les Brown.

*For those of you who don't know, in the "Dark ages" before camera phones and digital cameras became available, people used to take pictures with these shitty cameras that had a plastic reel thingy inside and you had to go to a studio to get pictures developed (Print the pictures off the plastic reel). Then you had to scan them if you wanted to send them to your friends. And there was no YouTube, Facebook, Twitter or Instagram. See what older people went through! No wonder people used to be pissed off all the time, lol.

But Romi, what do I do with "them" (the bullies/stupid people)?

It's sad but true there are going to be people who will make fun of you and call you names if you are fat. I can't stand these stupid people. I will admit I enjoy fat jokes too but I always offer advice to people to be fit and never ever do I make someone look bad in public. If someone is putting you down in public, it only means they are nothing but a "**little bitch**". They have low self-esteem and they need to put you down to feel better about themselves.

If you are in such a situation you can react in more than one way. You can chose to "get hurt", cry, get angry and fight back, not get affected or "**own them**" by using a funny comeback.

YOU HAVE FULL CONTROL OF HOW YOU FEEL. If you get hurt, it's your fault.

Remember this – other people's opinion is nothing but an opinion, it is not your reality, don't let their opinion affect your state of mind and cause stress. Nobody has any right to insult you, even if your lifestyle is unhealthy. Only listen to people who support you and uplift you in a positive way.

And if you are a goofball like me, have some comebacks ready, for example:

"You can fix fat, but you can't fix stupid" or something along those lines. This will teach them a lesson to not insult and disrespect others and make them think twice before they say something offensive again.

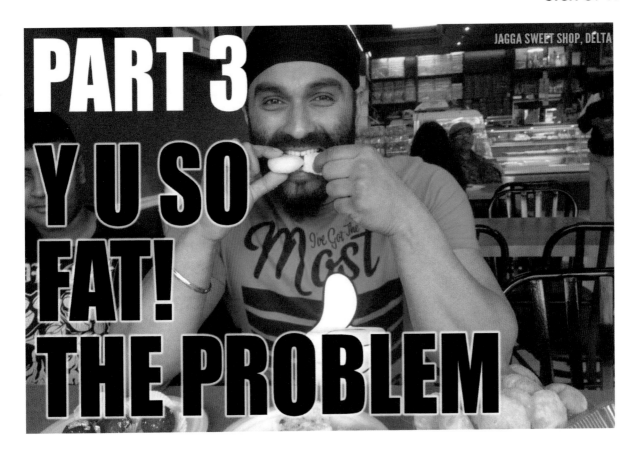

PART 3

Y U SO FAT! THE PROBLEM

JAGGA SWEET SHOP, DELTA

What comes to mind when someone asks you "Hey, why are out of shape"?

"Because my dog ate my healthy food". This excuse is legit, my puppy dog (A Maltese) actually eats my healthy food. He is very fond of broccoli and cashews.

Who gives a shit why you are fat?

It doesn't matter why you are fat. Stop worrying about excuses to justify your fat.

"Roses are Red, Violets are blue. You are Fat. Thank you."

Let's work on getting rid of it – **THE SOLUTION** and not the problem.

If you really want to know, then Google "Why am I fat?" You will get 630 million search results – go crazy "researching" the problem.

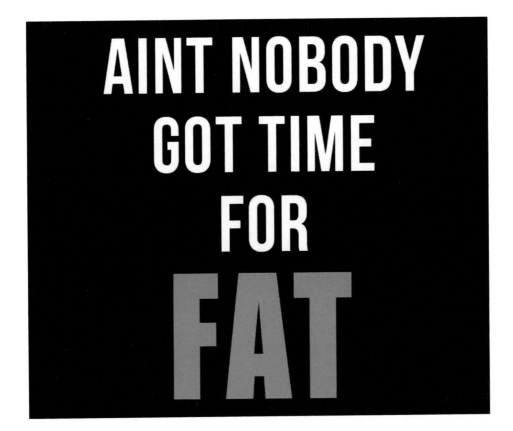

Excuses

Let's play a game...

List all excuses why you are out of shape and don't exercise and eat healthy...

You will probably come up with something like the list below,

But wait...

Let's make this fun. Read the list below and say "I hate this shit" after every excuse in comedian Chris Rock's voice. *Watch Chris Rock's YouTube video titled "Chris Rock – Love". Warning: He uses a lot of swearing and strong words in his video.

I don't have time, "I hate this shit"
Family responsibilities/kids, "I hate this shit"
I'm too tired, "I hate this shit"
I'm sick or injured, "I hate this shit"

My family isn't supportive, "I hate this shit"
The gym is too expensive, or too far, "I hate this shit"
It's too hard, "I hate this shit"
I don't know what to do at the gym or how to lose weight, "I hate this shit"
I don't know what to eat, "I hate this shit"
I'm not strong, fast, flexible, "I hate this shit"
I hate running, "I hate this shit"
The weather sucks (too cold, rainy, hot, etc.)., "I hate this shit"
I'm Lazy, not motivated, "I hate this shit"
I never got a pony for my birthday…, "I hate this shit"
I have to get up and go to my lame job everyday…, "I hate this shit"
I am a sweet potato.., "I hate this shit"
Romi it too busy to respond to my 10,000 questions, "I hate this shit"
..Blah blah blah…

Romi's cool new book.. "I hate…" errr HEY HEY HEY… "I love this shit!".

Remember, you LOVE this Book. Now go tell your friends to <u>go buy a copy</u>. Thank you!

Do you want to know **THE REAL REASON** why you are out of shape and don't exercise and eat healthy?

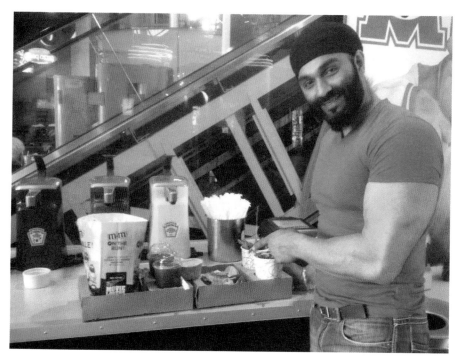

Because, like me, you love food and hate exercise.

You probably tried it all – exercise and diets and got sick of it.

QUESTION: Do you think that diets don't work?

FALSE! You are wrong. Diets work. "See Food diet", I eat everything I see. This diet which you follow has made you look this way. It works, haha.

One of my favorite comedians Lavelle Crawford (who I think is the best comedian ever, is really Fat, check him out on YouTube) said, "If I am going to eat this food, I might as well eat cardboard. Do I look like I follow diets well? Get your stupid ass out of here." This line is so funny it kills me every time I think about it, haha.

In my 13 years in fitness I have tried pretty much everything to get people to go on a healthy diet and a regular cardio program but I've always failed. People stop responding to my text messages. PS: I hate talking on the phone. Why call when you can text, right? Haha.

Do you know what happened with my clients who tried dieting?

Scenario 1

Every single client quit after a week or two while a few lasted a month. Then they went on a "See Food Diet". They binged and ate everything in sight and put on more weight than they lost.

But Why Romi, Why? You have such a lovely smile, why don't people listen to you?

People don't listen to me because our brain doesn't like giving up food (or anything for that matter). When we are forced to give up the foods we want, it only makes us want them more. When we are forced to eat healthy, our brain revolts. Try telling a kid not to play a video game and see what happens. This is like getting an arranged marriage like Indians used to, back in the day.

There was a lady at my old job, she said, "Romi, the Indian family across the street from us had 5 boys. 4 had arranged marriages and are living happily together. The youngest one who found his own wife was miserable and got divorced".

Moral of the story: get your family/friends to find you a husband/wife, lol.

OK fine, be like that, go find your own life partner. Let's get back to weight loss, shall we? Please stop distracting me.

This is what happens with diets at a mental level (psychologically). You try to give up all the good and bad foods that you had been eating and replace them with something tasteless, and you try to force every meal down your throat. Now you might not have an issue with this food otherwise but when someone tells you what to do, your little brain says, "I will show them" and makes you do the opposite.

Your life used to be so much fun and so comfortable, and now, all of a sudden you are forced to make friends with a treadmill or a track. Yet you try to do it.

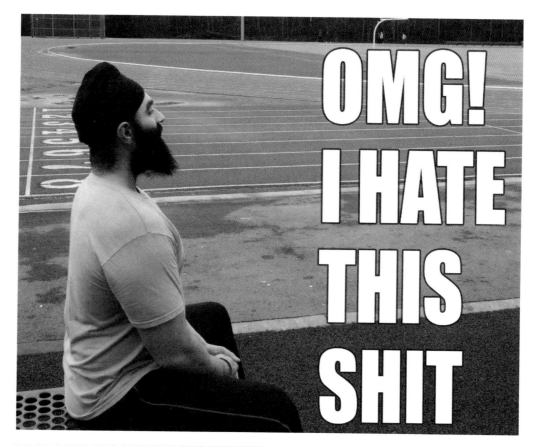

DON'T lie, admit it, this is exactly how you feel. I feel the same way about cardio. I did it anyway to look cute and sexy for you to have nice pictures of me to look at, for motivation of course, haha.

So, you try cardio. A few days go by and BOOM you snap. You can't take it anymore and you indulge in any food you can get your hands on – Ice Cream, Donuts, Pizza, cheesecake. You say to yourself, "we will do this diet and exercise thing some other time." You say profound quotes like, "You Only Live Once" and start going backwards.

End Result: You gain more weight than you started.

Note: I don't call fat people fat... when you gain weight, I call you what you are – "plump". My First Lady gained 10 lbs on her two month trip to India, I called her "my cute little Plump baby", I almost got dumped. For those who don't know she's 5 feet 10 inches tall and fit, and she trains almost every day (and we eat bagels every day after gym). Only thing that saved me was my big muscles, I mean love, and her high self-esteem. Thank you God for giving her such strong mind, haha. Man that was close. WOOOOOO.

Moral of the story: A man should be a man, ladies love men who are "Ballsy" (like the book written by my coach Melissa Kravichek – "Be Ballsy"). I mean be nice to your lady, if you don't want to be dumped lol.

Check out this other funny story involving my First Lady, before we move on.

You guys already know how much of a Jerk I am, I mean what a cool honest guy I am. So this happened before we started dating when we had just met.

A sweet lady Raj who needed help with teaching kids the Punjabi language introduced us to each other, and my First Lady is her niece. I was going to help her with the project. Raj runs a website called www.punjabiteacher.com.

My First Lady trained at my gym – Platinum Athletic Club, Surrey. It is the best gym in the Vancouver area. I started talking to her and since I always give advice to people about exercise, I gave her tips and pointed out to her, how she could get more out of exercise. She told me a story of how she got so busy with her business (she is a Fashion Designer) that she had no time to exercise and she gained 15 lbs. Then she told me how she worked out hard for 2 months and lost 15 lbs.

I looked at her and, in my usual sarcastic tone, I said, "ooh you lost 15 lbs, what you want a cookie?" lol. She shared this story with me afterwards. At the time she thought "OMG, what a Jerk. But at least he's an honest jerk".

I almost got dumped before even getting to know her, lol. But then again I have big arms and a hot body, I mean, she had me at "Hello".

To cut this story short, she likes me for my integrity, belief in God (#1 priority in life), and how much I care about people (especially her) and motivate them to improve in all areas of life. I had to work hard for 6 months to go from friendship to relationship, lol.

Let's get back to weight loss.

Scenario 2: By some divine miracle, you stick to your diet and lose weight in 2 months. You get compliments from everyone you meet and you are proud of your accomplishment. You feel like you are at the top of the world. You feel like Paris Hilton.

You want to rest and reward yourself with some time off and delicious food. 1 week of indulgence turns into one month, but you still look good and you don't have to worry about getting back to the gym. You say to yourself, "I will start my diet and exercise next week" and start procrastinating, and eventually you start resisting it.

You end up gaining weight and getting demotivated as you say to yourself, "What's the point, I tried and gained it all back again". You quit and end up gaining more weight than what you started with.

Now you create a belief that "I tried everything, and nothing works".

Remember that girl (who I mentioned in Introduction) that told me "What's the point of killing yourself in the gym if you can't eat what you want"?

Her comment made me change my attitude towards diets. I changed my diet and started eating the foods I wanted to (while I continued to train). I only followed strict diets for my bodybuilding competitions.

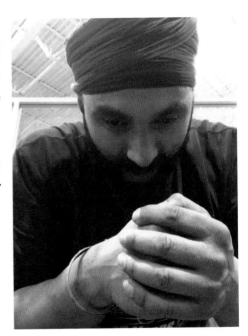

If you are thinking "OMG! I have no hope. I am going to die fat", don't worry, there's hope for you, and we will get you a bigger coffin.

Err, I mean Romi will get you in shape.

Read on my Fitness Warrior!

Part 4

The Solution

The Mighty Pillars of Success

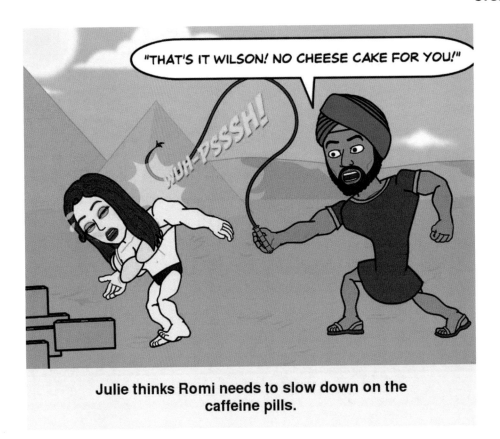

Julie thinks Romi needs to slow down on the caffeine pills.

I call my solution – "The Mighty Pillars of Success!"

This solution is The Mighty Singh's Mind & Body Training System. This solution fixes your mindset and allows me to "mind-control" you to become Healthy and Fit. I mean, it motivate you, there is no such thing as Mind Control.

This method shows you how to be in control of your mind and make the right decisions for yourself and not be a slave to others. Do it for you!

If you use the word "BOOORIINNNNGGGG" and "YAWWNNN", I will come over there and kick your ass. Just shut up and read on. I mean, Kindly read on my lovely Fitness Warrior, hehe.

Now that we have everything on the table, lets hold hands and sing, err, I mean let's focus on the solution that will keep you healthy, fit and happy for life.

You are guaranteed success, if you follow my advice.

In return I only ask for one thing. Whatever you learn from this book, please share it with as many people as you can. You never know who is going to relate to you and follow your advice or your lifestyle, and make a positive difference in his or her life. This is the whole reason I started sharing my progress. People started connecting with me and started making the right decisions to take control of their mind and their health.

Whoever you help, tell them to share what works in their life with others. This is my way of making this world a better place. BOOM!

Please follow every single step below, don't be lazy – you can read this while having cookies, cheesecake, pizza or any junk food of choice.

This method is guaranteed to work because it includes the success principles used by hundreds of motivational speakers, personal trainers, coaches and athletes.

These principles are slightly modified by me based on my life experience and my experience with clients who actually made a difference in their health and life.

PILLAR 1: Accept yourself and Expect Great things in life

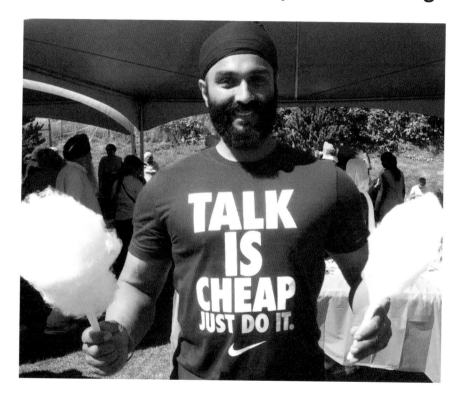

What does acceptance mean?

We all have strengths, weaknesses and ego. People have and people will always point out your weakness and rarely will they appreciate your strengths because humans love negative gossip.

Do this exercise or else I will come over and KICK your ass!

Before you accept yourself, take a piece of paper out and write down all of your weaknesses and strengths. Write all the good and bad things you do on a daily basis, even as small as opening a door for someone, and as bad as cursing someone in your mind.

This is your personal inventory. Look at all your strengths and pat yourself on the back (use your right hand and reach back of your left shoulder and pat it like a boss, haha).

Now look at your weaknesses and write down what triggers these bad things, anger, ego, low self-esteem etc. even if you don't show these emotions or feelings to others.

We need to eliminate these negative emotions, actions and reactions from your mind. Don't change anything, just observe your actions and notice what causes you to react or think in a negative way. For example, if someone posts a negative comment on your Facebook or Instagram or If they say it to your face. What is it that makes you think or say "F*ck you A$$h*le."

Now you know what you need to work on, accept yourself and love yourself for who you are as a person. Do not accept bad habits, bad health and fat.

There was a time in my life where I had Zero motivation, no motivation to eat healthy, exercise or do anything in life. I thought of myself as a loser and hated myself. I even gave up bodybuilding, which is something that I value more than anything. I had nobody to look up to, I went to God and he saved me via Spirituality. I finally started appreciating life and started helping others who were also in a stressed state of mind (which most people confuse with depression).

I don't care whether you believe in God or not – you should appreciate your life as a gift and love yourself. If you don't love yourself, you can't fully love and appreciate anyone else.

Believe in God but don't be an Asshole!

We only find solutions when we start asking questions. All of us have to fight our individual battles in our mind and win. Some people find their answers in sports. Others find answers in helping people in stress, while others find their answer in music etc. You need to find your answer.

This is not to be confused with ego and selfishness. Love yourself but don't be an asshole to others.

Never put others down (always uplift and help others) because negative comments affect most people, you don't want to be the cause of stress in their life. You don't want to be the cause of making someone's life miserable. If you can't add anything positive to other people's lives, keep your mouth shut.

<u>Expect good things in life</u> and have a strong desire to get what makes you happy. You should want it as bad as I want ice cream (and I absolutely love ice cream).

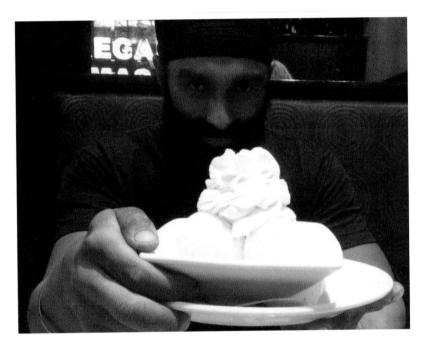

Accept yourself even if you are out of shape, stressed, depressed, down, in a bad relationship, in debt, or in any other bad situation. You have to love yourself to make a change. Remember, bad experiences teach us a lot – you have to make the decision to change your current situation and stop feeling sorry for yourself and stop expecting others to feel sorry for you.

Come on. Make that decision to make a positive change in your life. Do it.

EXERCISE:
Stand up. Put your hand on your heart and REPEAT AFTER ME:

"I love myself

I am going to be healthy, happy and fit"

^ Tweet that shit

PILLAR 2: You Need an Attitude Adjustment

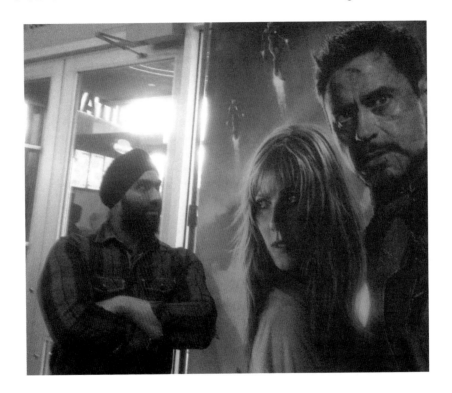

What is Attitude?

Your attitude is how you think, act and react towards yourself and others.

Negative self-talk (what you think constantly) and negative phrases you tell others to describe you or your habits are both destructive, and determine whether you are going to be happy and healthy.

If I had a cookie for every time someone said, "I don't exercise because I am lazy", I'd be a Cookie Monster!

Let me explain...

Eliminate negative words and phrases from your thoughts, your conversations, your messages and from your life such as, "unhealthy", "lazy", "weight loss", "fat loss", "I want to lose weight", "I want to be skinny". Erase these words from your mind. Cover your ears when someone uses these words.

Why should I avoid negative words and negative people?

Because these words program you negatively. Even though you are trying to negate these negative words, what you are really doing is training your brain to focus on what you don't want. When you repeat something over and over, it becomes your reality. Instead of becoming healthy, you will become fat and/or lazy and you will wonder why you can't motivate yourself. Instead of financial freedom you will find yourself getting deeper in debt.

ACTION: change your attitude from negative to positive.
Think positive thoughts and speak positively.

Stop talking about what you used to be - lazy, unhealthy, fat, in debt etc.

Replace "I don't want to be an asshole"

With "I want to be a good person, just like Romi"

Replace "I want to lose weight" with "I want to be Healthy, Happy and Fit" or

"I want to weigh X lbs in 2 months" or

"I want to be fit, lean, toned, be able play a sport, or run a marathon (whatever your goal is)."

This is called a positive affirmation. You need to tell you brain what you want, or want to change, rather than what you don't want. Don't even use the word "try", instead use "I am going to do so and so..." or "work in progress" because the word try is associated with failing. For example "I tried to eat healthy... but then I drove past a pizza shop."

Rome wasn't built in one day, neither was Romi.

PILLAR 3: Break free from the Prison of Negativity

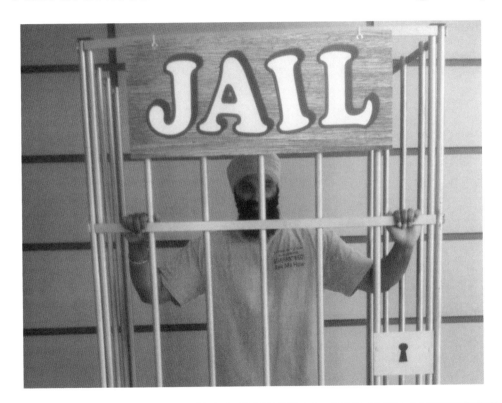

Do you think you are Free?

FALSE! You are a Slave!

If you check, you will realize you are a slave to your mind. Full of negative thoughts and limiting beliefs that you are constantly programmed with.

Your attitude is not wrong, it is just not in line with your goals and a happy life.

Just like we remove weeds from our garden to let grass grow, we have to constantly monitor and remove negative and limiting thoughts from our mind and replace them with positive thoughts, to move ahead in life.

ACTION: You should not do something because everybody else is doing it. Make your own decisions, set your own rules, and find your own way of doing things in life to accomplish your goals. Don't worry about what others think; do not live your life in fear. REMEMBER, Successful people are **WARRIORS** not Worriers.

There's always more than one way of doing things. Forget society's rules. Do what makes you feel good and come closer to achieving your goals. If you have not yet found success and are still doing the same things that you have always done, you will feel stuck and lose passion for your goals.

Break free, enjoy life, don't take life too seriously, be goofy, be silly, and have fun.

To be free and positive you can meditate, watch funny movies/shows, laugh, volunteer and help people. These activities give you a "natural high" because of a rise in "feel-good hormones" (levels of dopamine and serotonin) in our brain.

<u>To prove my point, I can get you super excited in less than 30 seconds.</u>

Go to YouTube and search "peanut butter jelly time" and play the first video that comes up.

Now you have "Peanut butter jelly time" stuck in your head.

Peanut butter jelly time…

Peanut butter jelllllllllly…

Peanut butter jelly, Peanut butter jelly, Peanut butter jelly
Peanut butter jelly, Peanut butter jelly, Peanut butter jelly

You get the point. Now go annoy someone else with this song, haha.

And YOU, my lovely fitness warrior, get back to this book. Let's move to the next step. OMG, keeping your attention on this book is like Dieting – Impossible!

PILLAR 4: Forget "Balance"

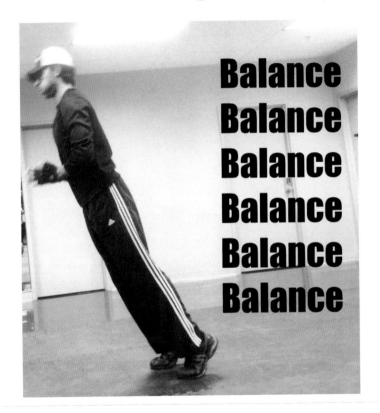

"You need to have balance", how many times have you heard this? The common belief is that if we focus too much on one thing, everything else must suffer. For example, while focusing on making money some people neglect health and relationships including family.

In the process of balancing everything you start stepping back from areas you excel in. This makes you mediocre in those areas as you become better at others. End result: you become mediocre at everything.

From observing successful people, failures and my own experience in life, I have learned that successful people have everything in life, health, family, happiness, money and peace. People who are not successful are always attempting to seek a balanced life and always complain about how miserable their life is.

Then what should I do?

Use **RomiMagic**!

According to **RomiMagic** principle, there are no limits to what you can achieve in life. The only limits are the ones you set for yourself. Focus on the good and eliminate all the limiting factors and you will be successful. BOOM!

ACTION: Follow the following steps to go beyond your limits:

1. Write, on a piece of paper, everything you want to accomplish (for health, fitness and other major areas)
2. Set a 2-month deadline and write down what you want to achieve in 2 months.
3. Be more productive and fill up your free time with activities that are in alignment with your goals.

PILLAR 5: Create more free time in your day

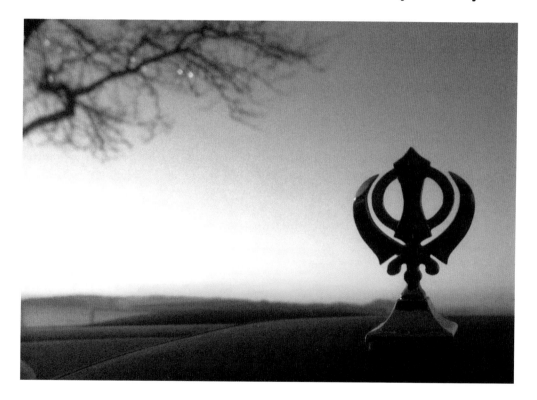

SAY BOOM if you agree: Who wants to free up more time in their day to do stuff?

Everyone has the same 24 hours in a day, yet successful people who are busy get more done in the same amount of time as the rest. I used to have long days full of different tasks both personal and professional and very little time to relax. One day I sat down and analyzed my schedule and figured out 3 main reasons we don't have time in the day.

Here's how you can be more productive and free up more time in your day:

1. **Plan, Plan, Plan:** You've heard the expression "failure to plan is planning to fail," haven't you? Without planning, we do things on the go without a schedule.

   Every night write a schedule for the following day with an estimate of how long it will take you to accomplish each item. Make this list on a small piece of paper, like a 3"x3" sticky note. (This is a well-known technique for time management.)

70 | P a g e

Then break the tasks down into components and cross things off when you have completed them. You will be amazed to see how productive you have been (and how much better you feel) when you see things crossed off your daily list.

2. **<u>Focus on what you are doing</u>**: You may pride yourself on being able to "multi-task" but in reality what you are doing is "task switching." You are not fully focused on an activity when you begin to focus on another and are not giving either of them the attention you should and can end up making mistakes or taking longer to finish both tasks. Only computers can truly multi-task, not the human brain. This does not mean you shouldn't take advantage of any unplanned downtime by tackling some of the smaller tasks on your list.

3. **<u>Don't expect downtime after finishing something:</u>** After working hard at your job, school, exercise, housework, etc., you think you deserve a "relaxing" break. Downtime makes you rush things you have to finish for the rest of the day causing you to make mistakes and sometimes redoing things over and over. A brief break is fine. Keep a timer handy when you take your small breaks and discipline yourself to get back to work or move onto the next task when that alarm goes off. Five minutes spent checking Facebook can easily turn into an hour (or more!) before you know it. You can take a long break when you have crossed off all the items on your to-do list and your new list for the next day is ready to go.

Implement these techniques and BOOM you've used all of your time well and have free time to do as you please.

PILLAR 6: Save some money and go on a Vacation

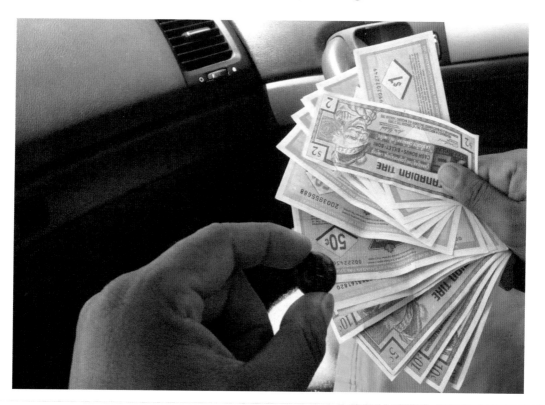

A lot of stress is our life is caused by lack of money or debt, therefore, saving money and eliminating debt will put your mind at ease.

Did you know if you cut 1 daily cheat meal, you can save over $2,500 a year?

1 fast food meal costs about $7 a day, which means $210/month and $2,520/year.

What can you do with extra $2,500? I don't know – maybe go on a vacation, buy a new phone or an electronic gadget.

If you don't want to go on a vacation, send me a cheque for $1,500 and save the rest. Oh come on, it's worth it; I will give you my blessings haha.

Now you have a positive mindset and you know what you want, i.e. you are under Romi's hypnotic spell. Be scared. Be very scared.

PILLAR 7: I hate Diets

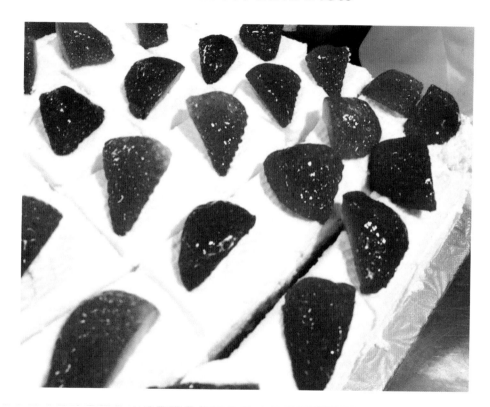

"The Mighty Singh's dietless plan"

Before I suggest a food plan, I want to add that if you are following a diet, and it's helping you get into the shape you want, continue what you are doing.

Also, there are several quick weight-loss network marketing companies with products that really work, if you want to use any of those, it's also fine as long as you get shit done.

"The Mighty Singh's dietless plan", is very simple, you are not restricted from eating foods you want. Here's what you do in this plan

1. Eat more food
2. If you don't want to eat clean, eat what tastes good
3. Have 3 big meals in a day, and one or two smaller meals
4. Eat fruits and vegetables with two of your meals
5. Space your meals. Give about 2-3 hours between meals
6. Protein shakes and smoothies are allowed as one meal
7. Do not limit your carbs, you need carbs for energy
8. Don't stress about calories and numbers
9. Do not eat foods that make you feel like shit
10. Drink lots of water throughout the day
11. Post pictures of your meals on Twitter/Facebook/Instagram

As a rule of thumb, try to eat at least 4 times a day. Eat somewhat healthy foods for breakfast and dinner. Find the time to have two or more meals in the day. The only condition is to make sure the meals are not too close to each other or too far apart, and don't eat anything between meals. If you feel like having ice cream or a slice of pizza with your meals go ahead, but make sure you have fruits or raw vegetables in that meal.

Eating this way will give you energy all day and you will not experience a crash and burn after half a day. When you only have 1 or 2 meals in a day, your body uses up some food and stores some food as fat because your brain knows you will starve your body by not eating enough and your metabolism slows down. With more food in your system your body keeps processing food and giving you energy (your metabolism speeds up).

The funny thing about frequent feeding is that your body eliminates excessive cholesterol and fat from your body. Eating fruits and vegetables keeps detoxifying your body to some degree (to do a full detox/cleanse check out my website for an article on a 3-day cleanse where you don't have to starve yourself).

Forget counting calories and worrying about other numbers, what's more important is to fix food timing and eating more meals. Focus on getting meals that fill you up. Counting calories and grams of protein, fats and carbs only adds more stress that you don't need. If you must measure, then do rough estimates, for example 1 cup of Broccoli (and don't put Cheddar cheese on it, it defeats the purpose of eating broccoli, lol). Also, you end up eating less than you need.

Benefits of this food plan:

1. You have more energy
2. You look sexy
3. You become healthy
4. You are less cranky and not mean to people
5. If you exercise/play sports you don't get tired easily
6. You have more stamina
7. You feel happy
8. You love Romi (Oh come on, you know you do, haha)

PILLAR 8: I HATE EXERCISE

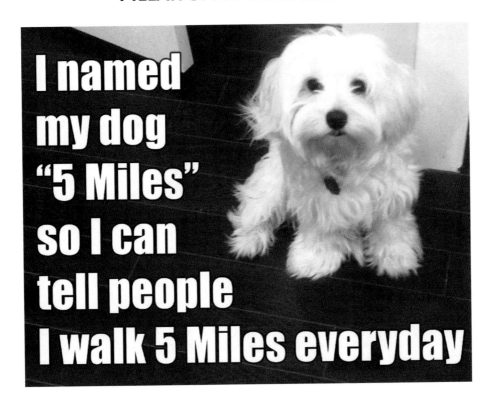

I named
my dog
"5 Miles"
so I can
tell people
I walk 5 Miles everyday

Why does Romi exercise so much?

Don't hate! I love exercise because:

- It makes me feel good
- The gym is my second home
- I love the pump that I get from weight exercises
- Sweating with cardio or sauna cleanses my skin and cools my internal organs because I am so hot ☺
- Keeps my immune system strong
- Makes me look sexy
- Gives me an opportunity to take pictures to post on Facebook and Instagram

Now, I am not saying you have to go to the gym to exercise. There are hundreds of ways to get exercise done.

Check this out for different ways to get exercise:

1. NO, Typing and texting on phone is not exercise, lol
2. NO, Eating food is not exercise for your jaw, lol
3. Go for a walk on the street, a park, a trail etc.
4. Go for a jog at the track
5. Play your favorite sport (NO, Nintendo/Xbox/PlayStation don't count, those are the sports that make your ass Fat, lol)
6. Go for outdoor physical activities like hiking
7. Join martial arts classes
8. Go for a bike ride (NO, motorcycle doesn't count, don't get cute with me OK)
9. Go swimming
10. Wash your car (already did it? Come wash my car, haha)
11. Clean your house
12. Go Rollerblading

13. Go dancing
14. Walk around the mall
15. Do pushups/situps etc at home while watching TV
16. Park your car far away from the mall or work, to get extra walking in
17. Take the stairs at work (unless you work on the 27th floor, lol)
18. Mow your lawn (or come Mow mine)
19. Go on a Picnic date with your special someone (if you are "forever alone" go alone, lol)
20. Do Yoga
21. Sit in a Sauna for 5-10 minutes (and please shower after)
22. If you have kids or a pet, play with them
23. Join a gym and do cardio or aerobics classes
24. Volunteer
25. Climb up and down the stairs

No matter what you do – make it fun. Take pictures, especially silly ones. Here's an example, Spiderman crunches, haha.

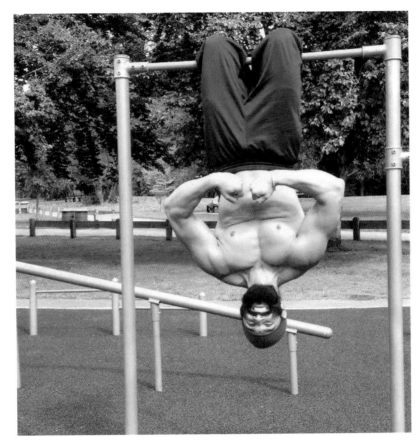

There are several other ways to get your heart rate up. Be creative, don't give me bullshit excuses "I don't know what to do to exercise."

Do something regularly about 3-4 times a week and you will keep your heart healthy. This will help you slowly lose weight, and you will lose inches first and then you will lose weight.

How to make training more exciting?

To make it easy and fun, find a training partner who also wants to become healthy and fit.

Announce your goals publicly to your friends and family and also on Social Media (Facebook, Twitter, Instagram etc). Making your goals public keeps you accountable and helps you keep moving to save yourself from public embarrassment.

If all else fails and you are still not motivated, simply imagine me and ask yourself **"What would Romi do?"**

Part 5 – Romi's life in pictures

My life is very exciting and stress-free, because I live my life by the rules I taught you in this book. Since pictures are the best way to tell a story I've added pictures of my life, which show you what I do every day and what I eat.

This is not a diet or exercise plan, this just shows you how I live my life. I will be publishing a detailed nutritional plan in my next book.

No matter what your situation is, make sure you have fun win life. Take a lot of pictures and say BOOM. Sharing pictures on social media websites inspires your friends to take care of their health.

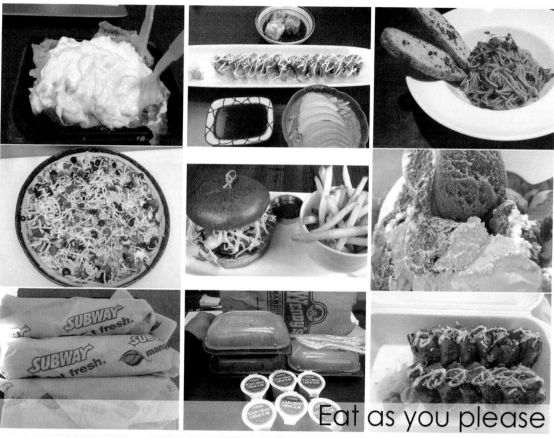

Eat as you please

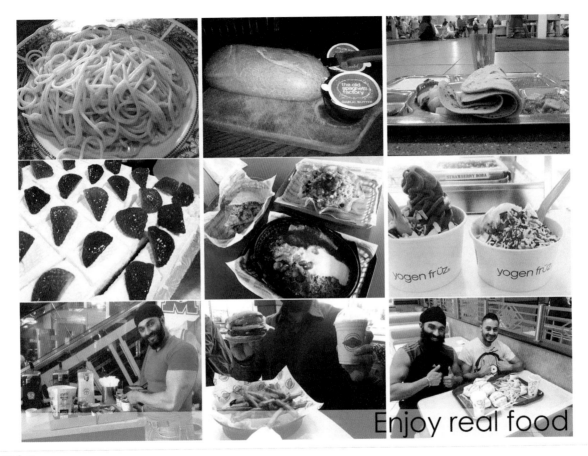

Enjoy real food

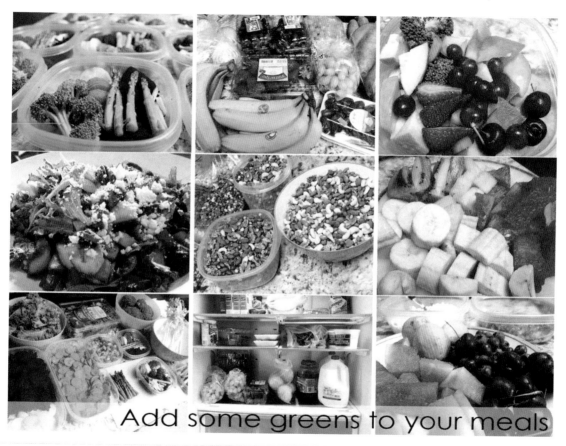

Add some greens to your meals

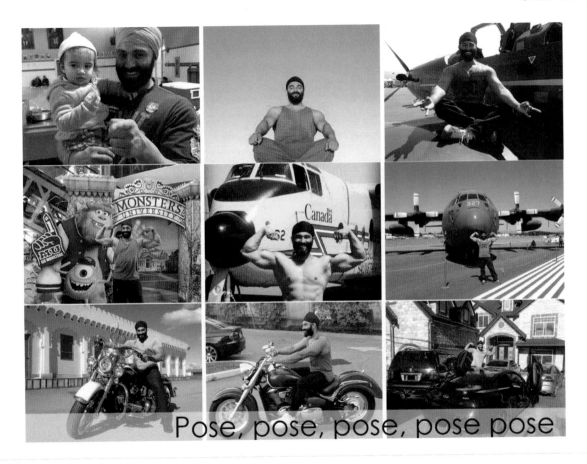

Pose, pose, pose, pose pose

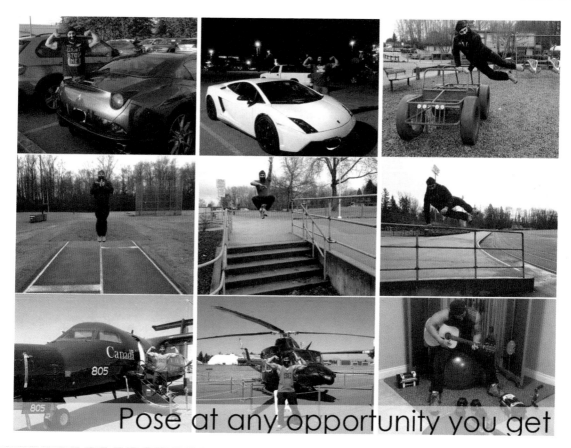

Pose at any opportunity you get

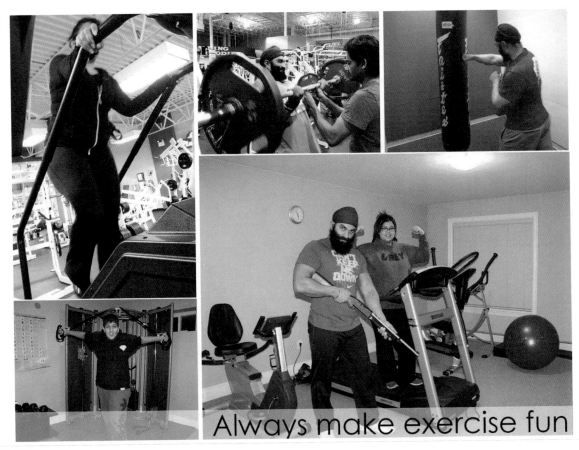

Always make exercise fun

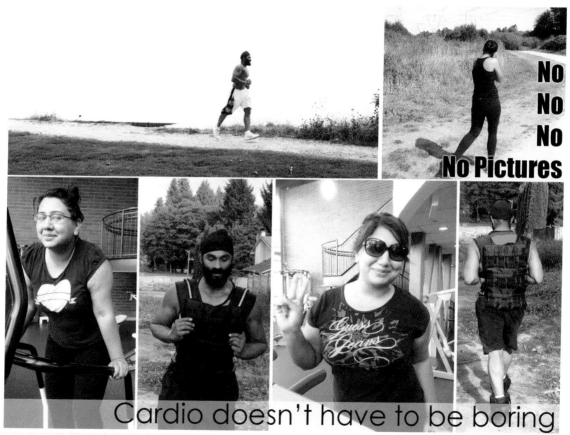

No
No
No
No Pictures

Cardio doesn't have to be boring

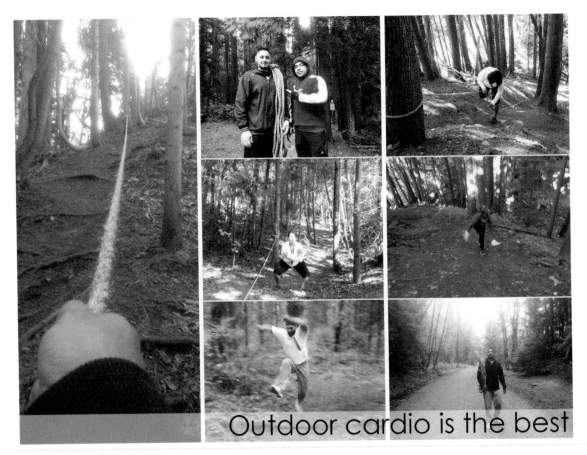

Outdoor cardio is the best

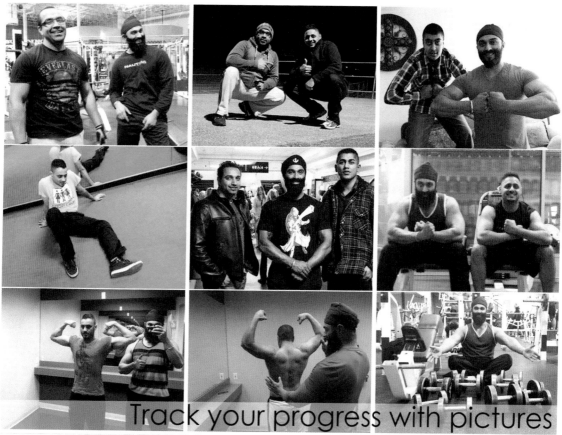

Track your progress with pictures

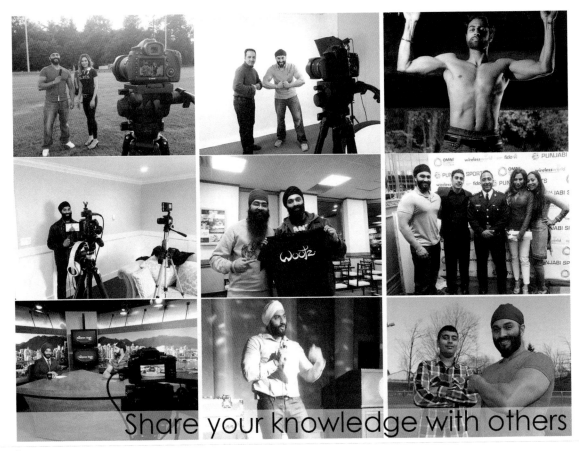

Share your knowledge with others

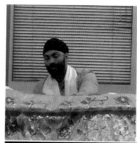
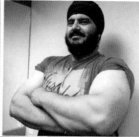

Big Thanks to my best friend Mander "The Tank" for training with me and being at the gym daily before all of my competitions.

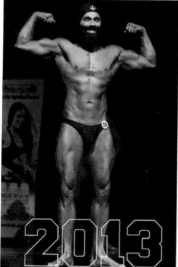
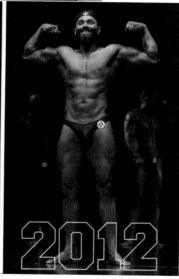
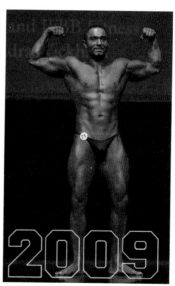

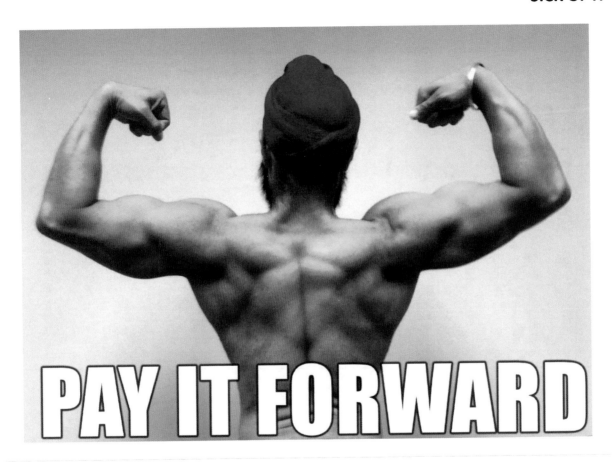

Paying it forward!

My request: If this book helps you make a positive difference in your life, please share what you have learned from me with your friends. And ask them to share it with others. I believe this is how we can make this world a better place – by changing one person at a time.

It would be nice if you recommend people buying my book, but if you think this book might help someone, lend this book to them.

Can I get a BOOM?

Next book

My next book will be about people who applied the principles laid out in this book and changed their life.

It will cover their stories about how their life was before and how they used The Mighty Pillars of Success to change their life.

Testimonials

"Romi, I am not sure if you still remember me. I see your posts on Facebook and get my son to read them too. He told me he sees you at the gym sometimes. I feel you are a great role model for a lot of people – especially the youth. We definitely need more people like you."

Polly

"Romi is an incredible young leader driven by a passion to help others grow, learn and become more confident through peak physical training and conditioning. His expertise in fitness and bodybuilding helps clients become comfortable and increase their level of stamina and endurance. Romi's professionalism, knowledge, skills, abilities, and talent is unmatched and the results his clients receive leave them coming back and wanting more. I HIGHLY recommend working with Romi one-on-one or online. His passion, enthusiasm, and charisma is contagious and will help you light a fire within. I can tell you from the thousands of dollars I've spent in gym memberships and trainers the results I've received won't compare. 7

lbs gone in 10 days with a few simple changes which included getting off my ass and working out and that's only the beginning. (Yes he can be tough) I couldn't ask for a better fitness accountability partner or inspiration. To many more successes and an incredible transformation!"

Melissa Krivachek, President, Briella Arion

"Romi has taught me to have faith in my own abilities. Watching his accomplishments have brought me strength in my own physical training. I started a proper diet and an exercise program due to heart disease. I can only say that my doctor has nothing but praise for the changes that I have made in my own life. Romi was an example of what hard work and a positive attitude can accomplish in your life. Thanks Romi for being an inspiration on my bad days and a "fan" of mine on my good days. You are the best!"

Joe Barnes, Journalist & heart attack survivor

"As a person and as a life coach Romi is a kind, caring, and optimistic gentleman. He shows his kindness through the respect he has for others' thoughts and feelings. He doesn't ever put you down he lifts you up. He is a great role model for all ages, especially the youth in our community. Through his motivation and determination that is seen on his Facebook page I have been able to make healthier choices in my life. Thanks Romi. Keep doing what you do. You are great at it."

Lakhi

"I have known Romi for about 4 years now. I came to know about Romi through a dear friend. I contacted him and told him about my desire to bring a change in my physique. A meeting was scheduled and Romi took control of everything from my diet to my weight training. During my first two months of training with Romi I added about 15 pounds of muscle to my frame. I had always believed myself to be a hard gainer and believed that I didn't have the right body type to gain muscle. Romi educated me on the various body types and told me that I was incorrect as in fact I had an athletic body type. The knowledge that Romi provided me increased

my self-confidence manifold and fitness became a way of life for me, a passion. I religiously practice eating healthy every day and avoid alcohol and any type of drugs. There are a lot of trainers out there but not a single one that will provide you with the knowledge and education so that you can eventually lead by example to others. Romi finds success when his students, clients achieve success. Romi is not there to empty your pockets but in fact bring about a positive change in your lifestyle and assist you in making you a more positive and healthier being. After being under the guidance of Romi in terms of fitness nothing seems impossible to me anymore."

TJ Gillan, Model and aspiring Actor

'Romi has helped me make better food choices and weight loss options through advice and great inspirational posts through his social media He's 100% all about natural food and weight loss supplements If I ever need advice or reassurance I call Romi Singh Gill (-:"

Tina Mackenzie

Get in touch with me

Email: romi@romigill.com

Website: www.romigill.com

YouTube: www.youtube.com/YourRightToBeFit

Facebook Page: www.facebook.com/CoachRomiGill

Facebook Personal Profile: Romi TheMighty Singh Gill

Twitter: CoachRomiGill

Instagram: CoachRomiGill

Made in the USA
San Bernardino, CA
26 February 2014